MW01026397

THE MOTHER OF ALL ANTIOXIDANTS

HOW HEALTH GURUS ARE MISLEADING YOU AND WHAT YOU SHOULD KNOW ABOUT GLUTATHIONE

BY JOEY LOTT

www.joeylotthealth.com

Publishing services provided by 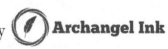 **Archangel Ink**

ISBN: 1517511798
ISBN-13: 978-1517511791

Table of Contents

4

The New Black

Glutathione is the new black. It's difficult to read *anything* about health these days without a mention of glutathione. And if we believe the hype, we might start supplementing with exotic-sounding supplements like liposomal glutathione, N-acetylcysteine, and biologically active undenatured whey protein, all in hopes that these supplements might make us invulnerable to sickness, rendering us practically immortal. Well, okay, maybe you don't necessarily strive for immortality, but avoiding unnecessary illness or healing from chronic illness sounds pretty good, right? And the hype would have us believe that glutathione can do that for us.

Hold on, though! Not so fast. Let's not blindly believe the hype. Instead, let's take a closer look and see if the hype is sound or not. That's what this book is about. Here are some of the questions I want to examine. What is glutathione and why might you care about it? Is more glutathione necessarily better than less? Are there appropriate or inappropriate times to elevate glutathione levels? If there are appropriate times, what are the safest, most reasonable ways to do so?

Before we get into the investigation itself, let me tell you how I came to learn about glutathione and how my skepticism evolved. A number of years ago, I became ill with Lyme disease, and it lingered for years. I was *extremely* ill—a matter I have written about in more detail in other books—and I experienced a strange ambivalence that is difficult to explain to anyone who has never experienced chronic illness. It needs little explanation to those who have suffered ongoing illness and the sense of defeat it engenders; I was simultaneously resigned to being bedridden and in an emotional and mental fog for the rest of my life *and* desperate for a solution.

Like many chronically ill people, that desperation led to *extensive* research. I read and read and read. At first, I read books written for the layperson, mostly intended for an audience of sick people desperate for a cookie-cutter answer to their ailments. After 20 or so of those books, I began to dig into primary sources such as medical research publications.

One of the things that I saw mentioned *over* and *over* again throughout my investigation was glutathione, and I'll admit to you that never *once* did it interest me enough to look into it and try to understand what glutathione is or what it does or why everyone seemed so keen on increasing glutathione levels. Frankly, there were hundreds of angles to look into, and glutathione just didn't stand out *to me* at the time. But I did note the frequent mention.

Fast forward several years. I had been enjoying improved health for several years when I moved into a rental house along with my family, including young children. The house was *extremely* moldy. I kid you not when I tell you that the 250-year-old stone foundation in the dirt-floor basement had an inch-thick layer of mold growth in places. When I and my children began to experience symptoms that I attributed to the mold exposure, I began to research the matter from various angles. Along with figuring out effective ways to reduce the exposure to mold (both spores and mycotoxins), I also wanted to find ways to detoxify any mycotoxins that we had ingested. The latter led me to glutathione yet again.

In fact, I read several studies that claimed that effective mycotoxin detoxification requires glutathione in the human body and that glutathione deficiencies are associated with mycotoxin-related illnesses. Finally, years after I had first started hearing about glutathione, I had what seemed like a good reason to actually begin to investigate the matter.

When I started to research glutathione, I found the primary literature on the subject to be *especially* dense. I'm quite accustomed to reading primary literature that makes most people's eyes gloss over as they drift off to sleep, so I'm no stranger to the usual density of these things. But the glutathione literature was initially impenetrable. The only *non*-technical terms in the papers were 'a', 'an', and 'the.' Otherwise, the rest of the words were things like 'peroxidase,' 'gamma peptide,' 'heterodimeric,' and 'gamma-glutamylcystein.' It took a

8

while before I started to understand, but little by little, I did.

As I started to understand the literature, what I kept thinking was, "There's something slightly fishy with the popular representation of glutathione." I couldn't *quite* put my finger on it, but something wasn't adding up. For example, I came across a lot of studies showing that glutathione levels in the body increase in response to potential toxins in some cases. One such example is a study that increased the levels of an oxidant called peroxynitrite[1] in cow heart cells and found that the increased *stress* led to an increase in glutathione production.

I found myself asking, "If glutathione levels increase in the presence of some potential toxins, might the common belief that more glutathione is always better be misguided?"

Unfortunately, I wasn't able to connect the dots to answer that question to my satisfaction. So in my initial draft of this book, I drew some useful, but ultimately *uninteresting* conclusions. Namely, I concluded that *adequate* glutathione levels are important, but *excessive* glutathione levels aren't necessarily better. Furthermore, after reading through the literature, I saw *few* legitimate needs for *most* of the common ways that people promote boosting glutathione levels. I did, however, offer some tepid support of some of the simple, reasonably safe, natural ways to maintain *adequate* glutathione at any given

---

[1] Buckley, B.J. and Whorton, A.R., "Adaptive responses to peroxynitrite: increased glutathione levels and cystine uptake in vascular cells," *American Journal of Physiology, Cell Physiology*, 2004;279(4):C1168-1176.

time—things like sleeping enough, a few gentle herbs with good track records, and adequate nutrition.

Although I say the conclusions weren't very interesting, it wasn't a *bad* manuscript. It was valuable in that it provided a more sober and balanced approach to maintaining health without falling prey to sensationalism and high-priced (and possibly even dangerous) supplements that are being promoted left and right these days. But still, something kept nagging at me. I felt that I wasn't doing the subject justice. So I sat on the manuscript for a while.

Then, fortuitously, I read a short piece published on the 180DegreeHealth blog written by Joel Brind, PhD, a professor of biology and endocrinology. Apparently, I was not the only to ask the questions I had been asking. In fact, the title of the piece written by Dr. Brind was "Glutathione: Is More Better?"

Dr. Brind filled in the missing pieces of information and confirmed what I had been suspecting. When it comes to glutathione, things are a lot more complex than is summed up by the prevailing meme that claims that more glutathione is always better. At the same time, while things are a lot more complex, the good news is that, in a practical sense, it's a lot *easier* than we've been led to believe. We don't need fancy liposomal glutathione supplements nor do we need synthetic glutathione precursor supplements like N-acetyl cysteine in order to be healthy *in most cases*. Instead, if we do a bit of sleuthing, we can find the weak links along the way and correct those. Generally, we can make those corrections with some simple and age-old advice such as sleeping more, eating enough, eating a balanced diet, getting some sun, and learning not to sweat the small stuff.

It's true, however, that in some cases, extraordinary circumstances may necessitate extraordinary measures in order to correct an imbalance. For example, as we'll see, there actually *are* some cases in which supplemental N-acetyl cysteine can be useful. In fact, it can even be lifesaving in some cases. However, for most of us most of the time, we don't need such extraordinary measures, and relying upon them may create an imbalance rather than restoring balance.

So with that introduction, let's next dig in and explore the interesting world of glutathione. We'll look at what is known about glutathione, we'll review some of the hype, and we'll sort fact from fiction. Along the way, we'll develop a sensible picture of how to best support health without relying on unnecessarily extreme or expensive measures.

What is Glutathione?

When the glutathione advocates explain what the heck it is and why we are supposed to care so much, they often refer to it as the "mother of all antioxidants." Now, of course, we're all conditioned to believe that antioxidants are always a good thing (and that more is better). We've been told that megadoses of vitamin C, for example, are a panacea that can cure everything from the common cold to cancer, and very few of us question these claims. So positioning glutathione as the "mother of all antioxidants" puts us into a receptive mode. We perk up and think, "Oh, hey, that sounds like something wholly benign and like it might be the thing that will help me to feel well (all the time)."

But let's pause for a moment and look to see what antioxidants are and whether having more of them is always a good thing. Antioxidants, as the name implies, are substances that prevent or stop oxidation. Oxidation is a process in which an unstable substance pulls electrons from other substances, creating other reactive substances called free radicals. For example, one theory holds that at least some types of cancer are the result of unchecked oxidation occurring in cells, [2] and it is generally accepted that oxidative stress can damage or kill cells and is involved in a wide range of injuries and diseases including not only cancer, but also Alzheimer's, cardiovascular disease, diabetes, and arthritis, to name but a few.

Now, obviously, if we oversimplify, it would seem that oxidation is bad and therefore antioxidants (those things that protect against oxidation) must be entirely good. Therefore, we may (mistakenly) conclude that taking more antioxidants is always a good thing. However, things are rarely that neat and *overly* simple.

The more that people study oxidation and the role of antioxidants in health, the clearer it becomes that it's much more complex than such a simple story would have us believe. For one thing, oxidation is not *always* a bad thing. In fact, there are many oxidizing agents (the things that produce oxidation) that are essential for human life. Take for example, the eponymous oxidizing agent: oxygen. Just about *every* high school student can tell you that we humans require oxygen to survive. Every cell in our bodies needs oxygen, in fact. And a person deprived of needed oxygen for more than five minutes may well die. But on the other hand, oxygen is highly reactive, and too *much* oxygen can actually kill a person due to oxidative stress.

---

[2] Khan et al., "Antioxidant enzymes and cancer," *Chinese Journal of Cancer Research*, 2010;22(2):87-92.

It turns out that there are *lots* of examples of oxidizing agents that are beneficial in the right amounts. For example, iodine is required to produce thyroid hormones, which are necessary to fuel energy production throughout every cell in the body. It's absolutely essential (in small amounts) but also a strong oxidizing agent, which is one of the reasons it is used to clean the skin or clean wounds. Another example is hydrogen peroxide, which the body produces naturally as part of the immune system in order to remove pathogens. Too little and you're in trouble. But on the other hand, too *much* hydrogen peroxide and you're *also* in trouble because it will start to damage your healthy tissue.

The *right amounts* of antioxidants are essential to keep the oxidative stress in check. However, *excessive* antioxidants can actually interfere with essential oxidative processes. This is a matter that is only now being studied, and that research is still in the early stages. However, already, some interesting information has come out in regard to the potentially negative effects of excess antioxidants. For example, several studies have shown that when antioxidant supplements such as vitamin C and vitamin E are combined with treatments to reduce arterial damage (usually statin drugs and/or niacin therapy) the antioxidants *reduce the effectiveness* of the treatment. Another example is that free radicals are apparently part of the body's defense system against cancer, and some research suggests that antioxidant

14

supplementation in cases of cancer may have detrimental effects.[3]

Another phenomenon that has been discovered is that supplementation with antioxidants is sometimes associated with an *increased risk of mortality*. This has been seen time and time again in epidemiological studies where populations that supplement with vitamins E, C, A, and beta-carotene have higher rates of all-cause mortality than those who don't. Obviously, epidemiological studies make it impossible to draw any conclusions as to *why* such a relationship exists. However, the relationship does exist.

One *possible* reason for the relationship between antioxidant supplementation and increased rates of death is that sometimes antioxidants can act as *pro-oxidants*. So ironically, excess vitamin C, for example, can actually result in *additional oxidative stress*.

"Wait a second," I can hear you saying. "What's the dealio? Are antioxidants good or bad? Should I get rid of my vitamin C and vitamin E supplements?" The answer is that it depends. Antioxidants are essential for health *in the right amounts at the right times*. And, in fact, numerous studies show benefits from antioxidant supplementation under *some* circumstances. For example, several studies have shown that modest selenium supplementation (selenium is considered to be an antioxidant) can improve some cancer outcomes. And vitamin C supplementation can be helpful in some

[3] Perera, R.M. and Bardeesy, N., "Cancer: When antioxidants are bad," *Nature*, 2011;475:43-44.

cases such as helping to reduce symptoms in diabetes. But increasingly the studies show that the story is *much* more complex than we've been led to believe. And indiscriminate supplementation with antioxidants with the idea that they will stave off sickness is misguided, given the evidence.

So now, what about glutathione? Is more glutathione always a good thing? Well, like all other antioxidants, it depends on the context.

Glutathione is the most abundant endogenous (meaning produced inside) antioxidant in the human body. Its importance in maintaining good health is fairly undisputed. And, in fact, low levels of glutathione are associated with a variety of disease conditions precisely because low levels of glutathione are associated with increased oxidative stress.

So on the one end of things, we have the possibility of low levels of glutathione (relative to excessive oxidizing agents and free radicals). That state is clearly not a great one, and in extreme cases it can even lead to death. However, the "more is better" and the "increase by any means" attitudes that are so prevalent fail to recognize the distinct possibility of generating *excess* glutathione. In fact, almost nothing is presently written about excess glutathione because the idea just doesn't even seem to fit into the paradigm from which most people are operating. However, as we'll explore in this book, there are reasons why more is not better.

The Structure of Glutathione

As mentioned previously, glutathione is the most abundant endogenous antioxidant in the body. The key word is '*endogenous*' because it turns out that, although extremely small amounts of glutathione exist in some foods, they generally don't survive the digestive process. So it seems fairly obvious that the body has a preference to produce and manage its own glutathione rather than relying on exogenous (produced outside) sources.

Although there are a few studies that demonstrate that oral ingestion of large amounts of exogenous glutathione *may* increase glutathione levels in the human body, most evidence suggests that oral supplementation of exogenous glutathione is not the most effective means to increase glutathione levels. Instead, at present, the general consensus is that the most effective way to increase glutathione levels is to increase endogenous production.

How does the body produce glutathione? This is a fairly significant matter to understand, as we'll see, because understanding the process by which glutathione is made (and renewed) can shed some light on understanding safe and effective ways to support the body's optimal production of glutathione without resorting to extreme measures that may create imbalances and negative side effects.

Glutathione is what is called a tripeptide, which is a fancy term that means that the glutathione molecule is composed of three amino acids. The three amino acids that make up glutathione are glutamine, cysteine, and glycine. The significance of these three amino acids is important, so let's take a look at each of them in a little more detail.

Glutamine is said to be one of the most abundant amino acids in animals, including humans. Glutamine is easily absorbed from dietary sources, and it is found, not surprisingly, in significant amounts in red meat, poultry, fish, dairy, and eggs. It is also found quite abundantly in grains, legumes, and many vegetables. In other words, a glutamine deficiency is extremely rare. For that reason, I have yet to come across any literature that suggests that glutamine is likely to be the limiting factor when it comes to glutathione production, and like most discussions of glutathione, in this book we will more or less ignore glutamine. (Though, considering that some people have problems with glutamine derivatives called glutamates, I do wonder if some of the benefits that some people experience by supplementing with cysteine derivatives come from the removal of glutamates from the brain.)

Cysteine is *generally* the focus of most discussions of glutathione synthesis. That is because it is generally thought that cysteine is the limiting factor in glutathione production. However, as we will see, I suspect that this view is only *partially* correct and that it misses some important points. In any case, understanding cysteine is going to be important for the rest of the discussion that follows in the book, so let's take a closer look.

When it comes to cysteine, the claim is that unbound dietary cysteine is poorly absorbed and can, in fact, be toxic in excessive amounts. Of course, some cysteine is essential for healthy functioning of the body, in part because it is required for glutathione production. However, it would seem that dietary sources of unbound cysteine are not the preferred way for humans to acquire needed cysteine.

Much of the marketing hype around glutathione claims that in order to increase glutathione production through cysteine supplementation, one must acquire a special form of cysteine called cystine (notice the subtle spelling difference), which is made when two cysteine molecules are bound together. In fact, reportedly, cystine is the form that is generally found in most *raw* foods. However, heat or acid treatment breaks the bond, a process called denaturing, which reduces cystine to two cysteine molecules.

So what are you to do? Should you start guzzling gallons of raw milk and parachuting raw egg yolks and liver? Well, you *could*, but it's not actually clear that that is necessary or even necessarily a great idea. While I once subscribed to the notion that raw foods provide health benefits, now I'm not so sure. In fact, there is some good evidence to suggest that cooking is one of the important contexts in which humans have evolved, protecting us from pathogens present in raw foods. So before we jump to conclusions, let's take an even closer look at the cysteine issue.

It is commonly believed among researchers that cysteine needs are higher in young children and in the elderly but lower in most adults. The implication is that the high levels of bonded cystine found in raw, human breast milk may be needed by babies, but the need for cystine in adulthood may be negligible. In fact, there is consistent evidence suggesting that elevated levels of cysteine in the blood have a linear, positive relationship with fatness.[4] In other words, more cysteine means more fat. This lends some credibility to the theory that cysteine is inflammatory and that excess may not be desirable from a health standpoint.

Again, adult humans do need cysteine. However, we only need a limited amount, and the evidence is that excesses are problematic—an observation that should be considered carefully before intentionally trying to increase cysteine levels in the body.

Humans produce cysteine indirectly from another amino acid called methionine. Methionine is considered an *essential* amino acid because the body requires it but cannot synthesize it. Like cysteine, methionine is necessary, but it is also inflammatory. In fact, numerous studies demonstrate that excess methionine is implicated in inflammatory disease conditions such as cancer, diabetes, and cardiovascular disease. This observation

---

[4] Elshorbagy et al., "Cysteine and obesity: consistency of the evidence across epidemiologic, animal and cellular studies," *Current Opinion in Clinical Nutrition and Metabolic Care*, 2012;15(1):49-57.

has given rise to a popular dietary approach of *restricting* methionine in order to prevent or reverse disease. However, while that approach in moderation may be healthy, as we'll see in a moment, it is possible that the same benefits may be had by *balancing* methionine intake with anti-inflammatory amino acids.

We'll look at the process by which the body converts methionine to cysteine in the next section because that is an important part of the puzzle. In fact, in my view, it is the piece that is overlooked by most people, and it is the key to understanding how to naturally support the body in achieving balance rather than overcompensating with cysteine and creating even more imbalance. For now, just know that there is good evidence that the adult human body is usually perfectly capable of meeting its cysteine needs *without* introducing large amounts of bioavailable cysteine

The final amino acid of our trio is glycine, which is one of the most abundant and yet least appreciated amino acids in the body. Glycine is considered non-essential, but that doesn't mean that we don't need it. Rather, that just means that it is *theoretically* possible to synthesize all the glycine that we need from other nutrients. As such, relatively little research has been done into the nutrient. However, some people are now estimating that many humans are now deficient in glycine by as much as ten grams per day.[5]

---

[5] Melendez et al., "A weak link in metabolism: the metabolic capacity for glycine biosynthesis does not satisfy the need for collagen synthesis," *Journal of Bioscience*, 2009;34(6):853-872.

In almost *every* discussion of glutathione, the potential significance of a glycine deficiency is overlooked, and in my view that is a major oversight. As we'll explore in subsequent sections, a glycine deficiency could *easily* be part of the reason why glutathione levels may sometimes be low while cysteine and cysteine analogs may be *elevated* in many people.

So there you have it. Glutathione is a tripeptide made of glutamine, cysteine, and glycine. Although I generally agree with the common consensus that glutamine is unlikely to be the limiting factor in maintaining a healthy glutathione balance, I disagree with the usual emphasis on supplemental cysteine and dismissal of the potential for glycine to be the limiting factor.

Homocysteine

In the previous section, we saw that dietary methionine may be one of the main sources of the cysteine that the body requires. Now, let's take a closer look at that process so that we can understand the possible weak links and the implications.

As mentioned, methionine is considered to be an essential amino acid because the body cannot synthesize it in sufficient amounts from other nutrients in most cases. However, methionine is a double-edged sword because, like cysteine, it is required for growth, but significantly less is required during adulthood. Excess methionine is inflammatory. In fact, methionine excess has been linked with many diseases.

The precise mechanisms by which methionine may be problematic aren't entirely known. However, when we examine the ways in which the body uses methionine, we begin to get a clearer sense of what may be going on.

Methionine is found in significant amounts in muscle meats (including fish), egg whites, grains, nuts, seeds, and, to a lesser extent in milk (in the whey) and some plant foods like beans. The World Health Organization estimates that adult human daily methionine requirements are approximately 13 mg per kilogram of body mass. That means that an 80 kg human needs around 1000 mg (or 1 gram) of methionine per day, though that amount can be even less if the diet includes other methyl donors such as betaine (found in beets and spinach) and/or dietary cysteine.[6] But in any case, the actual needs are quite low, and they can *easily* be met by eating moderate amounts of normal foods. For example, a cup of milk contains about 200 mg of methionine while two eggs contain 300 mg and a single hamburger contains 500 mg. So it's really rather challenging to eat a protein-sufficient diet that is deficient in methionine. However, plenty of people are eating an *excess* of methionine, meaning more than the body actually requires.

Now, once dietary methionine is consumed, the body has to do something with it. Methionine may get converted to a substance called S-adenosylmethionine, commonly known as SAMe (pronounced as "Sammy"). SAMe is known as a methyl donor because it is able to contribute a molecule known as a methyl group to processes in the body. Lots of reactions require methyl molecules, and so SAMe gets converted into homocysteine.

Now here is where it gets interesting because homocysteine, as the name suggests, is a cysteine analog.

[6] Fukagawa, N.K., "Sparing of Methionine Requirements: Evaluation of Human Data Takes Sulfur Amino Acids Beyond Protein," *Journal of Nutrition*, 2006;136(6):16765-16815.

And, in fact, homocysteine can be converted to cysteine in the body. We'll look at that process in just a moment because it's a significant piece of the puzzle. But before we do, let's look at what happens when homocysteine levels are elevated.

Elevated levels of homocysteine in the blood, a condition known as homocysteinemia, is associated with *elevated oxidative stress*, and that means that homocysteinemia is linked with lots of disease states. No one is positive whether homocysteinemia *causes* disease or if it is incidental, but the coincidence of homocysteinemia and disease is quite clear.

Under healthy conditions, homocysteine gets converted to either cysteine or it gets converted back into methionine, thus averting the potentially damaging effects of too much homocysteine. Let's look at how the conversion takes place.

In order for homocysteine to get converted to cysteine, several things are needed, namely glycine and vitamin B6. Then, of course, cysteine can be converted to glutathione if needed, which requires the addition of both glutamine *and more glycine*. If glutathione is not needed or to spare glycine (which may be insufficient), cysteine may be alternatively converted to taurine and sulfate. So a substantial amount of glycine is needed to fuel the conversion of homocysteine into something that is mostly non-toxic through the cysteine pathway, and additional glycine is needed to produce glutathione.

On the other hand, homocysteine can convert to methionine with the addition of vitamin B12 and folate, along with the methyl group they contribute.

Alternatively, a substance called betaine can also supply methyl groups to facilitate the conversion of homocysteine into methionine.

There is one more important factor that will determine the fate of homocysteine—the needs of the body. Hopefully, it is obvious that the body is intelligent, and so the decision to convert homocysteine to methionine or to cysteine or to alternatively allow for a buildup of homocysteine is not simply made willy-nilly. Rather, the decision is made based on *need* and availability of nutrients. What that means is that if the body already has an excess of either cysteine or methionine, we can reasonably expect that homocysteine may be diverted away from those pathways. The implication is that supplementing with *additional* cysteine may not be such a great idea if methionine and homocysteine levels are already high. Why? Because doing so may contribute to homocysteinemia.

Sensible Ways to Facilitate
Endogenous Production

If we accept that the body is intelligent and capable of maintaining health generally when given the right conditions, we might want to consider the implications of the preceding description of glutathione synthesis and the methionine cycle. Given that information, does supplemental cysteine actually seem like the most sensible approach *in most cases* for improving glutathione status?

In my view, supplemental cysteine is unlikely to result in *sustained* benefits, particularly if a glycine deficiency exists (or B vitamin deficiencies). Instead, it seems that cysteine supplementation will likely result in a further glycine deficiency and elevated homocysteine levels.

Simply based on the nature of the reactions necessary for the synthesis of glutathione and the methionine cycle, it seems to me that the nutrients that are most in need are B vitamins (in particular vitamins B6 and B12 and folate), as well glycine.

When it comes to vitamin B12, the *only* bioavailable sources of the nutrient are animal foods such as meat, dairy, and eggs. Those eating an omnivorous diet would have a very difficult time being deficient in B12. However, anyone who avoids animal foods or eats very small amounts of them is at risk of developing a deficiency.

Vitamin B6 is also found abundantly in animal foods, particularly meat. However, unlike B12, it is also found in a wide variety of plant foods. For example, beans, bananas, potatoes, sweet potatoes, avocados, and spinach are all excellent sources. So for *most* people, eating a balanced diet with a variety of fresh, minimally processed foods will provide adequate vitamin B6.

Folate, on the other hand, is a bit more difficult to come by unless you eat a *lot* of leafy green vegetables and orange juice or a fair amount of beans. In fact, many foods are fortified with synthetic folic acid because folate deficiency would otherwise be much more common. Unfortunately, there is evidence that many people (perhaps as many as 40 to 50 percent of the population) may have difficulty converting synthetic folic acid to the usable form of folate, which means that not only might folic acid supplementation be ineffective for many people to meet their folate needs, but it may actually produce some toxicity due to the body being unable to adequately process it. (However, toxicity likely only occurs in the context of *excessive* supplementation, and it is also not entirely clear that many people are actually *unable* to convert folic acid to an active form.)

You'll recall that I mentioned that betaine is yet another way in which homocysteine can convert to methionine. Betaine, as the name suggests, was originally found in beetroot, and beets are one excellent source of the nutrient. However, spinach turns out to be one of the very best sources of the nutrient. Betaine, also known as trimethylglycine (TMG), contains (as the name suggests) three methyl groups and a single glycine unit. So betaine supplies a *lot* of methyl groups and a little glycine. As we'll see in the next section, a lot of betaine can actually produce a methylation overload, so a little bit of beetroot and spinach may be good for you, but don't start drinking gallons of beet and spinach juice thinking that more is better.

The body can also synthesize betaine as needed from *choline*. Choline is found abundantly in egg yolks and liver, and to a lesser extent in cruciferous vegetables, fish, and spinach. Choline deficiency is associated with fatty liver deposits and homocysteinemia, so including choline-rich foods in the diet can help maintain (or improve) health in several ways.

As stated earlier, some researchers suggest that modern humans may often be deficient in glycine to the tune of 10 grams per day. So it seems likely that glycine may, in fact, be one of the most significant limiting factors when it comes to adequate glutathione synthesis.

Those who advocate for "ancestral diets" as an ideological dietary template are often quick to point out that, until very recently, it is likely that humans had much higher dietary intake of glycine and a relatively lower intake of methionine. And, in fact, recent studies do support the notion that the inflammatory effects of methionine are offset when balanced by adequate glycine.

Glycine is found in large amounts in the brain, skin, bones, connective tissue, eyes, and to a lesser extent other organs. It is believed that humans likely have historically had a higher glycine intake in part because they have traditionally eaten these glycine-rich parts of animals that are largely discarded today by most people. In fact, there is some evidence that one of the reasons that chicken soup has traditionally been considered to be a healing food is that it is made from the *whole chicken*, including the bones, connective tissue, and skin, which make traditional chicken soup preparations good sources of glycine.

Perhaps the most convenient way to increase glycine in the diet is by supplementing with free-form glycine, which is available as a nutritional supplement. However, for those who wish to be "pure," the most convenient modern food source of glycine is gelatin, which is generally about 20 to 30 percent glycine. That means that on average, it would require about 40 grams of gelatin to provide 10 grams of glycine in the diet.

In my view, based on the actual science, the most sensible way to provide the body with the adequate nutrition it needs to balance glutathione levels and maintain health is *not* to supply additional dietary cysteine as is normally advised. Rather, I think it is much more sensible to eat a diet that provides adequate vitamin B6, vitamin B16, folate, betaine, choline, and glycine. This can be done through a combination of whole foods, processed foods, and nutritional supplements. Doing so will support the conversion of homocysteine to cysteine as it is needed.

Vitamin B Supplementation

In the preceding section we saw how supplying adequate nutrients to support the conversion of homocysteine to either cysteine or methionine is a sensible way to support naturally healthy glutathione levels. We also saw that, in some cases, getting adequate B vitamins from food alone can be a challenge. So many people choose to supplement with B vitamins. However, considering the ways in which homocysteine is converted to either methionine or cysteine and considering the potential for toxicity of some types of B vitamins, the *forms* in which you supplement B vitamins *may* be potentially important.

The main B vitamins we've discussed are B6, B19, and folate. Each of these vitamins actually refers to a *group* of related substances. So, for example, folate can be in the form of folic acid, dihydrofolic acid, or tetrahydrofolate, to name a few. Normally, cheap supplemental B vitamins are provided in forms that are *not* biologically active but can be converted to biologically active forms *in theory* within the human body.

Again, take folate as an example. The most common form in which folate is provided in supplements is folic acid, which is *not* biologically active. In order for the body to use folic acid it must convert it into a usable form such as tetrahydrofolate.

The fact that non-biologically active forms of B vitamins must be converted to active forms has recently cast some suspicion on the efficacy and the safety of some supplements. In general, I suspect that these concerns are largely *over*stated and sensationalized, especially by those who stand to profit by selling biologically active supplemental forms of the vitamins (which are protected by patent). However, that doesn't mean that there's not some reason to be cautious when it comes to supplemental B vitamins. As I mentioned earlier, some studies have shown that as much as 50 percent of the population *may* have a difficult time converting folic acid to tetrahydrofolate, and that *may* sometimes result in toxicity.

So what are we to do? Obviously, the time-tested way to get nutrients is primarily from food. And that most likely remains the *safest* way to do so. However, there is also very good evidence that *many* people do *not* eat enough of some essential nutrients such as folate. And it seems sensible in those cases that a person would be much better off getting adequate nutrients from a supplement than not getting enough nutrients if he or she is unable or unwilling to get necessary nutrients from food.

If you are uncertain about how much of these nutrients you are getting from your diet, one simple way to track your nutrient intake from food is to use a service such as cronometer.com or fitday.com. These sorts of services cater to unhealthy food restriction obsessions, and so if you are easily trapped in restrictive mindsets, I advise that you use these services with caution. However, they are convenient (and interesting) tools for getting a sense of your nutrient intake. I suggest you use the free version of one of the services for a few days to a week just so you can get a snapshot that will give you a sense of how much of each of these important nutrients you are eating.

If you decide to supplement with B vitamins, I can make a few suggestions. First off, in general, it may be safer to use biologically active supplemental forms, but I'm not convinced that it is necessary, *especially* if supplementing with relatively small amounts. Most of the risks of toxicity come from very large doses of the nutrients. For example, the adult requirement for vitamin B6 is around 2 mg per day. When people supplement with 100 mg or more per day of the non-active form (pyridoxine) for many days, weeks, or months, they run the risk of developing toxicity which can result in nerve damage. However, note that 100 mg is *50 times* the amount needed. So to stay safe, you could simply supplement with *more reasonable amounts.*

With all that said, given the potential concern that some people may not convert non-active forms to active forms very well, using the active forms does offer slightly more assurance that you can actually use the nutrients that you are supplementing. Of these nutrients, B6 and folate are the two of most concern.

Vitamin B6 is most commonly available as pyridoxine, which is usually combined with something to form a compound such as pyridoxine HCl. That is the non-active form. The active form is a relative newcomer to supplements, and it is called pyridoxal 5 phosphate, or P5P. The P5P form is said to be safer even in larger amounts (though, again, I'm not sure it's generally advisable to use such large amounts).

There are several active forms of folate that are available. One is called metafolin, which is patented by the German company Merck (not to be confused with metformin, the drug). The other most common version is 5-methyltetrahydrofolic acid sold under the trade name Quatrefolic by the Italian company called Gnosis. There may be others as well that I am not aware of. In any case, both of these forms of folate already contain methyl groups, which means that they can *increase* methylation in the body, a subject that we'll look at in just a moment. Also, I'd advise against supplementing with more than 400 mcg of folate unless you have a very good reason to do so. And, furthermore, *if* you supplement with folate, it is also generally recommended that you *also* supplement with B12 *because* folate can mask B12 deficiencies which can eventually lead to serious health problems.

Lastly, if you are vegan or simply eat very little of foods containing B12 and *if* you refuse to include more dairy, eggs, and meat in your diet, you really should consider supplementing with B12. And you really should consider a glycine supplement (they are generally vegan friendly). Vegans *consistently* have elevated homocysteine levels,[7] and that is most likely due to a combination of B12 and glycine deficiencies. B12 supplements come in lots of different forms. I'm not convinced that it matters a whole lot which form you choose. The cheapest and most common form is cyanocobalamin, which *may* not be a great form primarily because it isn't active, though I haven't read much suggesting that the body would have a difficult time converting it to an active form. It also contains insignificant amounts of cyanide, which, though insignificant, one might as well avoid. But in a pinch for anyone who is B12 deficient, cyanocobalamin is far superior to *no* cobalamin. The other common forms are methylcobalamin, hydroxocobalamin, and adenosylcobalamin. Of those, at least in the United States, methylcobalamin is the most common, and it should be fine most of the time, but also be aware that it contains a methyl group, which can increase methylation, a subject that we'll look at next.

---

[7] Elmadfa, I. and Singer, I., "Vitamin B-12 and homocysteine status among vegetarians: a global perspective," *The American Journal of Clinical Nutrition*, 2009; 89(5): 1693S-1698S;

Bissoli et al., "Effect of vegetarian diet on homocysteine levels," *Annals of Nutrition and Metabolism*, 2002; 46(2): 73-79.

Waldmann et al., "Homocysteine and cobalamin status in German vegans," *Public Health and Nutrition*, 2004; 7(3): 467-472.

Methylation

Methylation is a hot topic these days. A lot of people are pushing a genetic angle, suggesting that many people (maybe 60 percent or more of the population) have genetic mutations that supposedly interfere with methylation, and so a lot of people are getting genetic testing done and finding out that they have one or more of these mutations. Those who believe in methylation defects claim that it means that such people need *more* methyl groups than others in order to be healthy. I'm not so convinced that this phenomenon works as many claim that it does, though there may be some truth to it. But in any case, too many methyl groups can be as problematic as not enough, and in today's methylation-crazed atmosphere, it's easy to become "over-methylated."

Methylation is a process of one substance donating a methyl group to another substance. Methylation has been reported in many processes in the human body. For example, we already saw how a methyl group is donated by SAMe to another substance in order for

SAMe to convert to homocysteine. For homocysteine to convert to methionine, another substance such as methylcobalamin (an active form of vitamin B12) or betaine has to donate a methyl group. But methylation has also been seen in the formation of and degradation of so-called neurotransmitters like dopamine and serotonin. So methylation seems like a fairly important thing.

Now there are a lot of people, *especially* those trying to solve problems related to autism and other distressing conditions, who are into methylation *big time*. They supplement with methyl donors like active forms of folate, methylcobalamin, and betaine (TMG) in order to try and "improve" methylation in the body, which they think may be *under*performing in those cases. They *may* be right, but whether they are or not, that does not *necessarily* translate into "everyone who experiences some health problems should supplement lots of methyl donor nutrients" because *over*-methylation can be as much of a problem as *undermethylation*.

The reason I mention all of this is that, when it comes to glutathione, methylation obviously plays an important role, and while enough it is important, too much can be very unpleasant and even harmful. If you refer back to our earlier discussion about the methionine cycle, you'll recall that methylation takes places at two points—the conversion of SAMe to homocysteine and the conversion of homocysteine to methionine. So you need adequate methyl donor nutrients such as active folate, methylcobalamin, and/or betaine. However, let's consider what can happen if methyl donor nutrients are available *in excess.*

If there are too many methyl groups, *particularly* when an excess of methionine is already present, then either homocysteine can build up *or* homocysteine will be converted to cysteine *and deplete glycine reserves.* So *over-*methylation can result in a worsening of glycine deficiency. The result can be problems with skin, bones, teeth, joints, cognition, and mood. So be careful about supplementing with active B vitamins and betaine (TMG) in the case of a glycine deficiency.

One obviously sensible thing to do in order to maintain healthy methylation in the presence of methyl donor nutrient supplementation is to ensure adequate glycine either through gelatin or a glycine supplement. Another sensible thing to do is to also include a small amount of niacinamide (a non-flushing form of vitamin B3) along with the methyl donor nutrients. In circles where people try to increase methylation, they often use niacinamide to reduce over-methylation symptoms. In their view, niacinamide (or any form of vitamin B3) "mops up" methyl groups. I'm not sure that's true, however. Instead, it could simply be that adequate vitamin B3 supports normal energy production and therefore prevents *excess* methylation.

The cautions in this section generally don't apply to those who are not supplementing with active forms of B vitamins or betaine. However, because a lot of people *are* supplementing with these things, I think the caution is warranted. If you are experiencing symptoms such as irritability, anxiety, insomnia, nausea, headaches, joint pain, or muscle soreness and you are supplementing with methylcobalamin, active folate, betaine, or large amounts of beet and spinach juice, *you may be experiencing the symptoms of overmethylation* which *may* be due to glycine deficiency in part. So try increasing your glycine intake either with gelatin or a glycine supplement. A niacinamide supplement may help as well.

The Pitfalls of Common Advice

Now we've looked at what would seem to be the most sensible ways to improve glutathione status naturally. How does that compare to the common advice available from most sources? Let's take a look.

Normally glycine is viewed as completely irrelevant. However, as we've seen, glycine actually plays several crucial roles in the synthesis of glutathione. So in my view, the common lack of interest in glycine is a major oversight.

Instead of emphasizing glycine and B vitamin nutrition, more commonly the advice is to supplement with cysteine. There are two ways in which we are generally advised to do this. One is through a synthetic supplement called N-acetyl cysteine (NAC) and the other is with foods containing (supposedly) bonded cystine, which theoretically survives the digestive process and can be used by the body to make glutathione.

Supplemental NAC *can* be a powerful way in which to quickly increase glutathione *in an emergency situation*. In fact, NAC is commonly used in emergency rooms to treat acetaminophen (paracetamol) poisoning. Acetaminophen poisoning depletes liver stores of glutathione *as well as* cysteine levels. Because of that, acetaminophen overdose can damage the liver and in severe cases can even lead to death. The standard treatment is to use intravenous NAC in order to recharge both cysteine *and* glutathione levels. It is notable, however, that glycine alone also can protect against acetaminophen damage. [8] Furthermore, NAC combined with glycine may be even more effective than NAC alone.[9]

Supplemental cysteine in a bioavailable form, whether from NAC or some other form, undoubtedly has beneficial applications in some contexts. However, given the information that we have explored in this book, I don't think there is a strong case to be made for supplementing with cysteine in most contexts.

Furthermore, most of the forms of cysteine that are marketed as increasing glutathione levels are suspect in my view. Here's why. For one thing, even in *unheated* proteins such as raw milk or raw egg yolks, theoretically, the highly acidic environment of the stomach would denature the bonded cystine, making it unavailable to an adult human. I haven't been able to find any literature that explicitly states as much, but I believe there is a good

---

[8] Vance et al., "Effect of glycine on valproate toxicity in rat hepatocytes," *Epilepsia*, 1994;35(5):1016-1022.

[9] Kon et al., "Role of apoptosis in acetaminophen hepatotoxicity," *Journal of Gastroenterology and Hepatology*, 2007;supplement 1:S49-52.

chance that most cysteine in food is *not* available for glutathione production. It is also interesting to note that the pH of human stomachs from shortly after birth until 2 years is *higher* (meaning less acidic) than those of humans older than 2 years. The implication is that breastfeeding infants may be able to absorb cystine that is *not* denatured by the digestive process. This would lend credence to the notion that cysteine in a bioavailable form is only needed in relatively large amounts by very young children.

But even if we are to allow for the possibility that some cystine might be absorbed in a usable form by adults, upon investigation, it seems to me that there is almost *no* chance of products such as so-called undenatured whey protein actually containing undenatured cystine. Here's why. Cystine is said to denature at anything above 105 degrees Fahrenheit. But *every* commercial whey product of which I am aware is made from *pasteurized* milk, including ImmunoCal and Proserum, both of which boast that they are undenatured and biologically active. Pasteurization *always* occurs at temperatures significantly higher than 105 degrees Fahrenheit. So honestly, it seems practically impossible that these products are what they say they are.

Admittedly, my test is only n=1 (actually it's n=4 because my kids and my partner are also involved), but my family has gone through a couple of pounds of Proserum whey protein concentrate, and I cannot detect any change. Given the pH of the stomach and the fact that the milk was pasteurized, I cannot see any reason why the whey protein concentrate would appreciably increase cysteine levels in the body *except* by way of increasing methionine intake.

Now, of course, if a person was genuinely methionine deficient, then supplemental methionine or something like NAC could improve cysteine status. But for the rest of us *most of the time*, I think they are unnecessary.

The other piece of advice that is commonly offered, especially by those that market glutathione products, is to supplement with something called *liposomal* glutathione. Liposomal glutathione is exogenous glutathione in which very small particles are wrapped up in a fat in order to trick the body into absorbing it. Some people even make their own liposomal glutathione to save money by purchasing reduced glutathione and placing it in an ultrasonic cleaner along with some lecithin.

Liposomal glutathione really does seem to increase glutathione levels. But the question that seems obvious is, "Is it a good idea?"

Given what we've learned, it seems to me that tricking the body into accepting exogenous glutathione—something it normally seeks to avoid—may not be so wise. Perhaps in an emergency situation it *could* be useful, but in the long run, daily supplementation with liposomal glutathione seems shortsighted. Here's why. For one thing, as we saw from the beginning, more glutathione, like any antioxidant, isn't *always* a good thing. For another thing, what are the implications of adding so much exogenous glutathione? I'm not sure anyone knows entirely what the full implications are, but we can guess at some of them.

Given the process by which endogenous glutathione is normally produced, I highly doubt that exogenous supplementation would shut down endogenous production *in the long run*. However, in the short term, all that glutathione may suppress the endogenous production, which could lead to a buildup of homocysteine.

All in all, the common glutathione "wisdom" seems shortsighted. While some of it may be appropriate and useful in *some* contexts, it simply doesn't seem all that wise for most of us most of the time.

An Ounce of Prevention

There's another important aspect to glutathione levels that is often overlooked in the rush to market miracle products. That is the value of prevention in keeping glutathione levels in balance.

Included in the long list of things that deplete glutathione are many environmental pollutants, both synthetic and naturally occurring, such as pesticides,[10] benzene,[11] and formaldehyde.[12] Benzene is found in petroleum products such as gasoline. In fact, filling stations are among the strongest sources of the pollutant. But benzene is also found in tobacco smoke as well as many glues, adhesives, paints, and other

---

[10] Krieger, R., *Handbook of Pesticide Toxicology, Two-Volume Set: Principles and Agents,* Academic Press; Second edition (October 17, 2001).

[11] Wiemels et al., "Modulation of the toxicity and macromolecular binding of benzene metabolites by NAD(P)H:Quinone oxidoreductase in transfected HL-60 cells," *Chemical Research in Toxicology,* 1999; 12(6): 467-475.

[12] Levovich et al., "Formaldehyde-releasing prodrugs specifically affect cancer cells by depletion of intracellular glutathione and augmentation of reactive oxygen species," *Cancer Chemotherapy and Pharmacology,* 2008; 62(3): 471-482.

substances frequently found in homes, making indoor air the second leading source of benzene exposure for most people. Formaldehyde is also found in tobacco smoke as well as many building materials such as particle board, plywood, and fiberboard. Formaldehyde is also used in many glues and adhesives, permanent-press fabrics, and even some cosmetics and personal care products.

Many drugs produce glutathione depletion. One of the drugs that is most infamous for depleting glutathione is acetaminophen[13] (also known as paracetamol or by the brand name Tylenol), as was mentioned earlier. Other pharmaceutical drugs may also deplete glutathione levels, though most are not well studied in this regard. And alcohol[14] is another drug well known for its ability to deplete glutathione.

Some dietary practices are capable of reducing glutathione levels, including calorie restriction, low-protein diet,[15] and veganism.[16] Also, diets containing lots of mycotoxins, such as can sometimes be found in

[13] Slattery et al., "Dose-dependent pharmacokinetics of acetaminophen: evidence of glutathione depletion in humans," *Clinical Pharmacology and Therapeutics*, 1987; 41(4): 413-418.

[14] Viña et al., "Effect of ethanol on glutathione concentration in isolated hepatocytes," *Biochemistry Journal*, 1980; 188(2): 549-552.

[15] Ling, P.R. and Bistrian, B.R., "Comparison of the effects of food versus protein restriction on selected nutritional and inflammatory markers in rats," *Metabolism Clinical and Experimental*, 2008; 58(6): 835-842.

[16] Krajcovicová-Kudláčková et al., "Alternative nutrition and glutathione levels," *Cas Lek Cesk*, 1999; 138(17): 528-531.

poorly processed peanuts and grains, likely contribute to glutathione depletion.[17]

Lifestyle practices that produce stress in the body can also deplete glutathione. Among the most common are insufficient sleep[18] and overexercise.[19]

Obviously, you cannot avoid all of these things. But you probably can do something about some of them. For example, you could choose to forego the acetaminophen or at least substitute another pain reliever that is less potentially harmful. You could reduce alcohol consumption. You could make sure to eat a calorie-sufficient, protein-sufficient diet. And you could sleep enough and avoid overexercise. In the next few sections, we'll look at a couple of these matters in more detail.

---

[17] Emerole et al., "The detoxification of aflatoxin B1 with glutathione in the rat," *Xenobiotica*, 1979; 9(12): 737-743.

[18] Everson et al., "Antioxidant defense responses to sleep loss and sleep recovery," *American Journal of Physiology*, 2005; 288(2): R374-R383.

[19] Turner et al., "Prolonged depletion of antioxidant capacity after ultraendurance exercise," *Medicine and Science in Sports and Exercise*, 2011; 43(9): 1770-1776.

Dietary Restriction

There are a variety of ways in which people may restrict their diets that can be detrimental to glutathione levels. In this section, we'll explore calorie restriction, protein restriction, and carbohydrate restriction in regard to glutathione.

Calorie restriction is popular for a variety of reasons, including weight loss and lifespan extension. Unfortunately, it is a poor strategy for both purposes, a matter I have discussed at length in other books. Unfortunately, calorie restriction is so commonplace and rampant these days that many people have a distorted view of what calorie sufficiency is.

Insufficient caloric intake in the extreme is clearly associated with reduced glutathione levels. What is not clear is what the cutoff is, since no human trials have investigated at what point calorie restriction produces glutathione depletion. However, given information that I have presented in other books, it is reasonable to suspect that even modest calorie restriction, when sustained for long enough, will produce glutathione depletion.

As I have demonstrated in other works, calorie restriction in humans, even a modest restriction allowing for 2000 calories a day, has been shown to lower thyroid hormone levels and increase stress responses, all of which can increase oxidative stress. It is reasonable, therefore, in the absence of evidence demonstrating otherwise, to assume that glutathione may be depleted under such circumstances since it will be used to reduce the increased oxidative stress.

Unless and until proven otherwise, it seems prudent to consume adequate calories on a daily basis. Based on research I have presented elsewhere, it seems that the minimum daily calories for adults is greater than 2000 (since 2000 calories a day in the Biosphere 2 experiment resulted in lowered metabolic rate and lowered thyroid hormone levels) and likely in the 2500-3500 calorie range.

Protein restriction is associated with lowered glutathione levels. Protein restriction may be intentional or unintentional. Many vegans and other people who are trying to be healthy unintentionally restrict their dietary protein intake. Therefore, if you eat little meat, eggs, or dairy and you are concerned about your glutathione levels, you may want to monitor how much protein you eat on a daily basis. Most recommendations suggest that 0.8 grams of complete protein per kilogram of body mass is what is necessary on a daily basis in order to avoid frank protein deficiency, and many dieticians recommend 1 gram of protein per kilogram of body mass even for low-protein diets. That means that a 160 pound (73 kg) person needs to eat nearly 60 grams of protein each day to avoid protein deficiency.

Protein deficiency can deplete glutathione levels in several ways. For one thing, insufficient protein intake may worsen an existing glycine deficiency, which we've already seen may be the weak link in most cases anyway. For another thing, protein deficiency can increase oxidative stress. So eating *sufficient* protein, including *modest* amounts (13 mg per kilogram of body mass) of methionine, is generally advisable for health.

It is worth noting, however, that when it comes to protein, more is not necessarily better. Remember that excess methionine could create an inflammatory burden in the body, so excessive methionine intake in particular is not advisable. In other words, those who are eating 12-ounce steaks for lunch and dinner may want to ease up a bit. However, given the glycine deficiency that most people are probably facing, increasing glycine intake may be beneficial across the board.

Carbohydrate restriction is also a popular dietary strategy, but it may lower glutathione levels if carbohydrate restriction is taken too far. Adequate insulin responses are necessary in order to help maintain healthy glutathione levels in part because insulin is what helps to move amino acids where they are needed. Although some amino acids do provoke an insulin response, carbohydrates are a more reliable way to achieve the effect. Therefore, it is sensible to eat some carbohydrates with proteins. Very low carbohydrate diets are also known to reduce insulin sensitivity. So eating moderate amounts of carbohydrates can help to maintain insulin sensitivity and to produce an insulin response adequate to help support glutathione production.

Otherwise, when we look at dietary factors that influence glutathione levels, it is worth noting that nutrient deficiencies can increase oxidative stress in the body while nutrient sufficiency can spare glutathione. This is yet another reason *not* to eat a restrictive diet, because the more varied and inclusive your diet, particularly if we're talking about real foods such as dairy, eggs, meat, fruits, vegetables, starch, and so on, the greater the likelihood of your meeting your nutritional needs.

Moderate intake of naturally-occurring antioxidants from *real food* (versus supplements) can spare glutathione as well. That includes the relatively small amounts of vitamin C, vitamin A, vitamin E, and selenium that are found in foods like butter, liver, eggs, fish, meat, and fresh fruits and vegetables. It also includes the *extremely* small amounts of plant chemicals such as polyphenols[20] that are found in fruits and vegetables—things such as quercetin found in red onions and apples, resveratrol found in grapes, catechins found in tea and peaches, and

---

[20] Biswas et al., "Curcumin induces glutathione biosynthesis and inhibits NF-kappaB activation and interleukin-8 release in alveolar epithelial cells: mechanism of free radical scavenging activity," *Antioxidant & Redox Signaling*, 2005; 7(1-2): 32-41; Alidoost et al., "Effects of silymarin on the proliferation and glutathione levels of peripheral blood mononuclear cells from beta-thalassemia major patients," *International Immunopharmacology*, 2006; 6(8): 1305-1310;Pandey, K.B. and Rizvi, S.I., "Protective effect of resveratrol on markers of oxidative stress in human erythrocytes subjected to in vitro oxidative insult," *Phytotherapy Research*, 2010; Suppl 1: S11-4.

rutin found in oranges and cranberries. These polyphenols and other substances found in fruits and vegetables are often isolated or synthesized and sold as miracle supplements in ridiculously large amounts. However, while they may exert strong, drug-like effects in that fashion, mounting evidences suggests that in such large amounts, they may create imbalances. It may be much better to simply eat *small* amounts from fresh foods as part of a varied and inclusive diet. Megadosing, even in the form of vegetable juices, may be misguided.

Rest and Activity

Adequate quality sleep is one of the most overlooked essential components of good health. So much so, in fact, that I have written an entire book on the subject, in part to persuade people to make sleep a priority. Along with all the other things that adequate sleep can do, it can replenish glutathione levels and prevent glutathione deficiency. It also seems that improving glutathione status can improve sleep, [21] creating a positive feedback loop of health.

For a more detailed study of the benefits of sleep and ways to improve sleep, see my book with the clever title, *Sleep*. In the meantime, know that human adults appear to require between seven and nine hours of sleep every single night. Less sleep than is needed causes health problems that will continue until the sleep debt is paid off. Furthermore, the natural, in-built circadian rhythm of the human body dictates that sleep is best during the

[21] Singh, et al., "Oxidative stress and obstructive sleep apnoea syndrome," *Indian Journal of Chest Disease and Allied Science*, 2009; 51(4): 217-24.

hours of darkness, and wakefulness is best during the hours of light. Bright light exposure during the day is important, and avoidance of bright light in the evening is also important.

If you wish to improve your glutathione status, adequate sleep is essential. Begin to make sleep a priority and set aside adequate time for sleep every evening. If you are tired, you probably need more sleep.

Although we are often reminded that exercise is good for us, unfortunately, we are rarely (if ever) reminded that different types of exercise have different effects and that while some types may promote health, others are harmful. When it comes to glutathione levels, some types of exercise can increase glutathione levels while other types of exercise can deplete glutathione.

Generally, we can divide exercise into low intensity and high intensity. Low-intensity exercise such as walking may contribute to maintaining healthy glutathione levels, but if so, that is not well understood. But in any case, it doesn't hurt when done in moderation. However, when it comes to high-intensity exercise such as running or lifting heavy things, the duration of the exercise makes a huge difference.

Sustained high-intensity exercise such as long distance running can create oxidative stress and even DNA damage in humans. [22] These are signs of glutathione depletion. On the other hand, high-intensity

---

[22] Briviba et al., "A half-marathon and a marathon run induce oxidative DNA damage, reduce antioxidant capacity to protect DNA against damage and modify immune function in hobby runners," *Redox Report*, 2005; 10(6): 325-331.

exercise performed in short bursts with adequate rest can lead to increased glutathione levels.[23]

Essentially, the evidence suggests that sustained cardio workouts such as long-distance running, elliptical training, and so forth may deplete glutathione levels while interval training for short durations can lead to long-term increases in glutathione levels. Importantly, however, adequate rest must be provided between workouts, which generally requires that workouts be limited to half an hour every other day at most.

---

[23] Bogdanis et al., "Short-term high-intensity interval exercise training attenuates oxidative stress responses and improves antioxidant status in healthy humans," *Food and Chemical Toxicology*, 2013; 61: 171-177.

A Practical Approach

In this book, we've covered a lot of information. Hopefully we've done so in a way that clears up a lot of the confusion about glutathione and separates the hype from the facts, giving you a *practical, simple, and safe* approach that you can use to maintain healthy glutathione levels without resorting to extreme measures or expensive (and potentially ineffective) supplements. Now that we've reached the conclusion of the book, let's recap and see how the findings from this book can be applied.

To begin with, it seems that the likely weak link in the glutathione synthesis process is not cysteine. Instead, it may be the nutrients vitamin B6, vitamin B12, folate, and glycine. Therefore, it seems sensible to attempt to obtain these nutrients in one's diet to prevent the bottleneck that may be happening with homocysteine.

For most people eating a varied, omnivorous, calorie-sufficient diet composed *mostly* of real foods (versus industrially produced food-like products), vitamins B6 and B12 should be easy to obtain. Folate may be more challenging, particularly if it is true that some people cannot convert synthetic folic acid (added to many fortified foods) adequately to the active form. Eating more folate-rich foods such as orange juice and leafy green vegetables *may* provide adequate folate. Otherwise, a *modest* supplemental folate (which some recommend should be combined with supplemental B12 to avoid masking a B12 deficiency) might be appropriate.

When it comes to glycine, the best food source is gelatin. However, if it is actually true that most people are short on glycine to the tune of 10 grams per day, that would require 40 grams of gelatin to make up for the difference. Frankly, I bet that when a diet is lower in methionine, the actual glycine requirements are probably lower, but I don't have any proof that is so. In any case, for those who cannot or will not eat much gelatin, supplemental glycine may be a good consideration.

All of this, of course, should be occurring within the context of a varied, calorie-sufficient, nutrient-sufficient diet. So unless you have very good reason to do so, restricting any macronutrient or food group is probably ill-advised.

Additionally, you can spare glutathione by sleeping enough and avoiding overexercise. Hitting the gym five times a week and sleeping six hours a night can ramp up oxidative stress, deplete glutathione stores, and put you into a chronic stress state that no amount of NAC, undenatured whey protein, and liposomal glutathione will fix.

Finally, it would seem that for most of us most of the time, the most sensible and healthful approach to maintaining balance is a moderate approach. The obvious answers that our research has provided may not be exotic or exciting, but they are probably much more grounded and *honest* than most of the glutathione hype. Sure, in emergency situations, extreme measures may be appropriate in the *short term*. But on a day-to-day basis, the tried-and-true basics of eating enough, sleeping enough, and resting enough are your best bet.

May you enjoy good health as you sidestep the dubious marketing claims of the supposed glutathione miracle...and the next "miracle cure" after that.

Get My Future Books FREE

If you enjoyed this book (Hey, if you made it this far it couldn't have been that bad), you'll probably enjoy many of my other books about health and wellness. And you can get all my new releases in health and wellness for free by signing up for my mailing list at www.joeylotthealth.com. It's simple, it's free, and it's totally honest and legitimate. Nothing scammy or spammy or anything else like that (i.e. I won't be trying to sell you The 7 Dirty Underground Top Secret Weird Tricks for Rock Hard Abs or Young Living Oils). It's just about free books for those who appreciate my work, because I appreciate YOU. Simple as that.

Connect with Me

I welcome your questions, comments, and feedback of any kind. Please feel free to email me at joeylott@gmail.com. I am now receiving so many emails that I cannot always reply to every email. I do read them all, and I do my best to reply to as many as possible. For the benefit of others, I may choose to publish my response to your email on my blog or in book format. I will maintain your privacy and anonymity if I choose to publish my response.

One Small Favor

My sincere goal in writing is to share something that may be of value to you. And I endeavor to do so while keeping the costs low for readers. The success of my books and my ability to reach other readers who may benefit from my books depends in large part on having lots of thoughtful, honest reviews written about my work. You would do me a great favor if you would please take a moment to generously write a review of this book at Amazon.com. This will only take a few minutes of your time, and you will be helping me a great deal. I sure would appreciate it.

About the Author

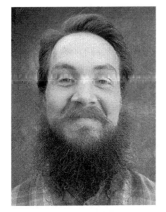

"The secret to happiness is to let go of everything - see through every assumption."

Beginning at a young age Joey Lott experienced intensifying anxiety. For several decades he lived with restrictive eating disorders, obsessions, compulsions, and an inescapable fear. By the time he was 30 years old he was physically sick, emotionally volatile, and mentally obsessed with keeping any and all unwanted thoughts and experiences at bay.

At this time Lott was living on a futon mattress in a tiny cabin in the woods. He was so sick that he could barely move. He was deeply depressed and hopeless. All this despite doing all the "right" things such as years of meditation, yoga, various "perfect" diets, clean air, and pure water.

Just when things were at their most dire, a crack appeared in the conceptual world that had formerly been mistaken for reality. By peering into this crack and underneath all the assumptions that had been unquestioned up to that moment, Lott began a great undoing. The revelation of this undoing is that reality is utterly simple, ever-present, seamless, and indivisible.

Lott's books provide a glimpse into the seamless, simple, and joyous nature of reality, offering a glimpse through the crack in conceptual worlds. Whether writing about the ultimate non-dual nature of reality, eating disorders, stress, disease, or any other subject, he offers the invitation to look at things differently, leaving behind the old, out-grown, painful limitations we have used to bind ourselves in suffering. And then, he welcomes you home to the effortless simplicity of yourself as you are.

Not sure where to begin? Pick up a copy of Lott's most popular book, *You're Trying Too Hard*, which strips away all the concepts that keep us searching for a greater, more spiritual, more peaceful life or self.

Made in the USA
Las Vegas, NV
18 December 2024

14454218R00039